W9-CZK-631

MAGGIE EATS HEALTHIER
by Paul M. Kramer

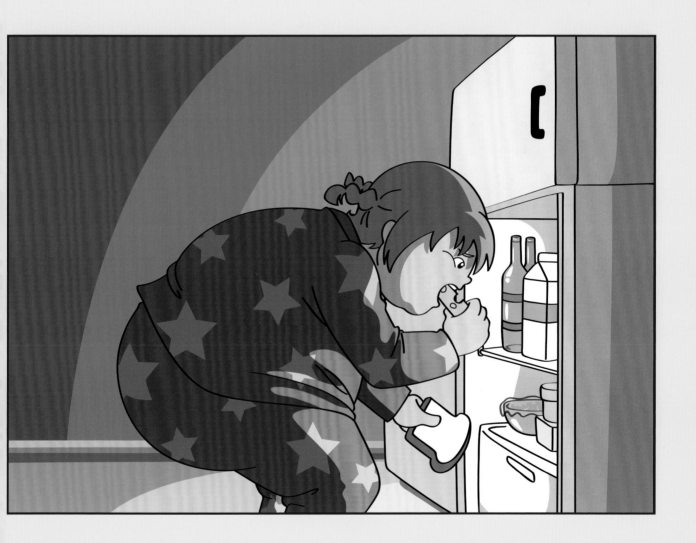

Maggie Eats Healthier by Paul M. Kramer

© Paul M. Kramer October 2014. All Rights Reserved.

Aloha Publishers LLC
848 North Rainbow Boulevard, #4738
Las Vegas, NV 89107
www.alohapublishers.com

Inquiries, comments or further information are available at, www. alohapublishers.com.

Illustrations by Mari Kuwayama greenwing001@hotmail.com.
Audio by Charly Espina Takahama charly@pmghawaii.com
Collaborator, Co-Editor, Cynthia Kress Kramer

ISBN 13 (EAN): 978-0-9827596-7-7
Library of Congress Control Number (LCCN): 2011960086
Printed in Guangzhou, China. Production date: September 2014 Cohort: Batch 1

MAGGIE EATS HEALTHIER
by Paul M. Kramer

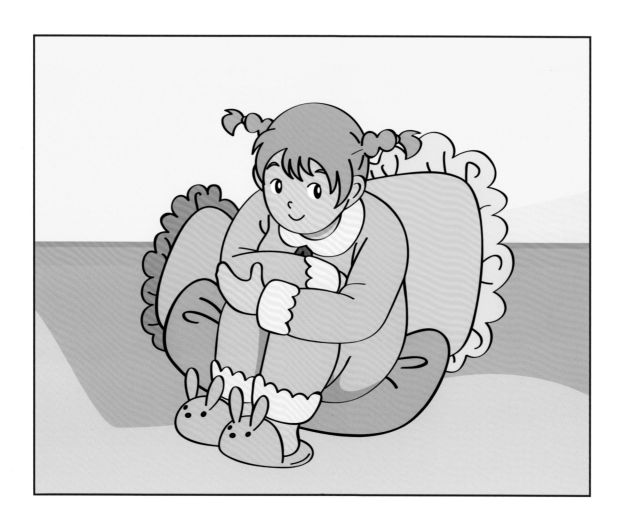

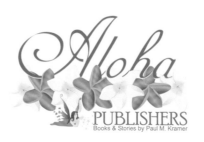

Aloha

PUBLISHERS

Books & Stories by Paul M. Kramer

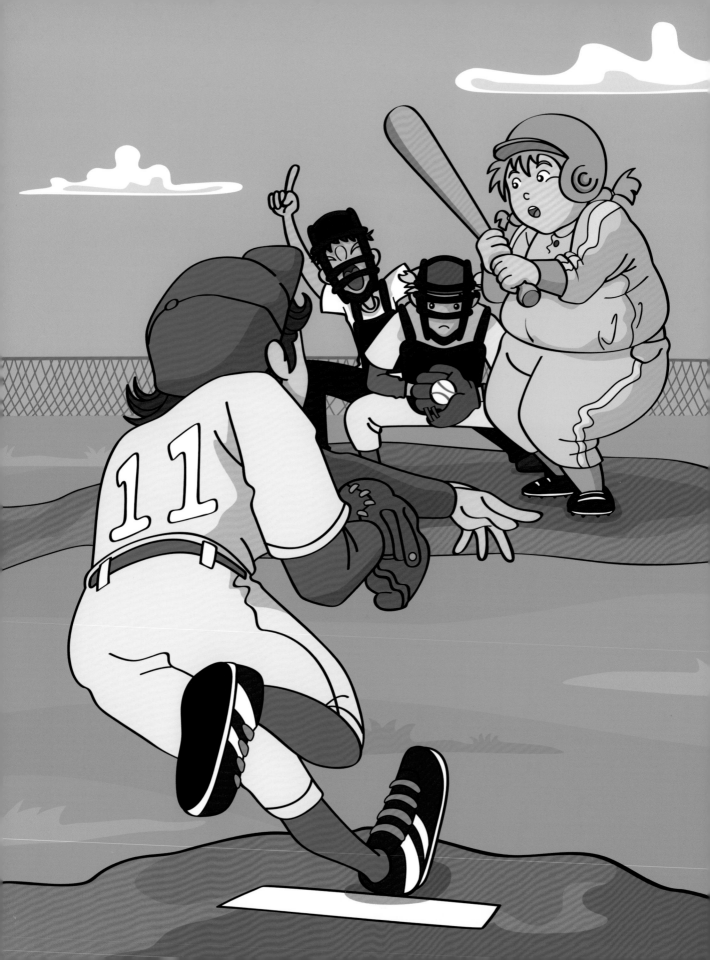

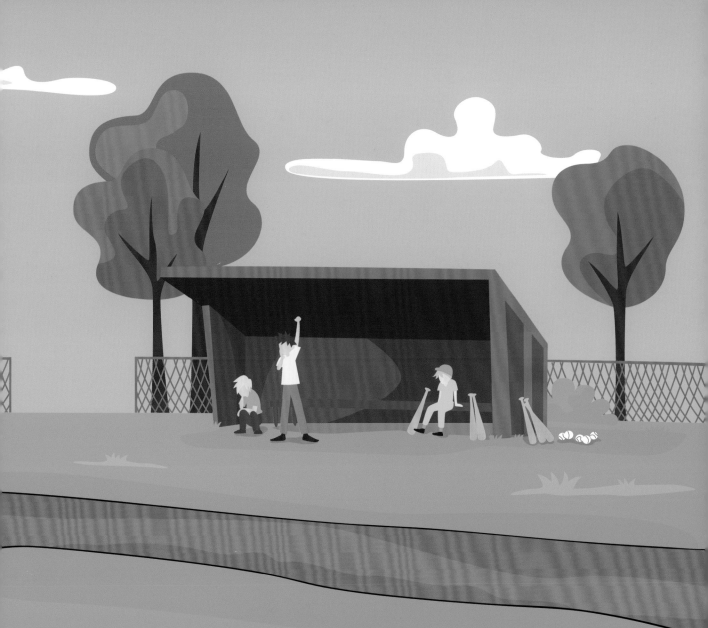

Maggie Magee loved playing sports but had not yet developed
athletic skills.
She had the desire and she had the will.

Sounds of chuckles were heard as Maggie got up to bat.
Maggie was already insecure without the added pressure
of being laughed at.

Disappointed in herself for she was the worst on the team,
Maggie was determined to one day be fit and be lean.

She couldn't understand why some kids could be so mean.

After the game ended Maggie was quite sad.
It was one of the worst days that Maggie ever had.

Anxious and depressed and not thinking clearly,
Maggie was holding on to her dignity, but only just barely.

Searching the refrigerator in hopes she'd feel better,
munching on bread and cheeses, especially cheddar.

Maggie was not going to allow anything else to upset her.

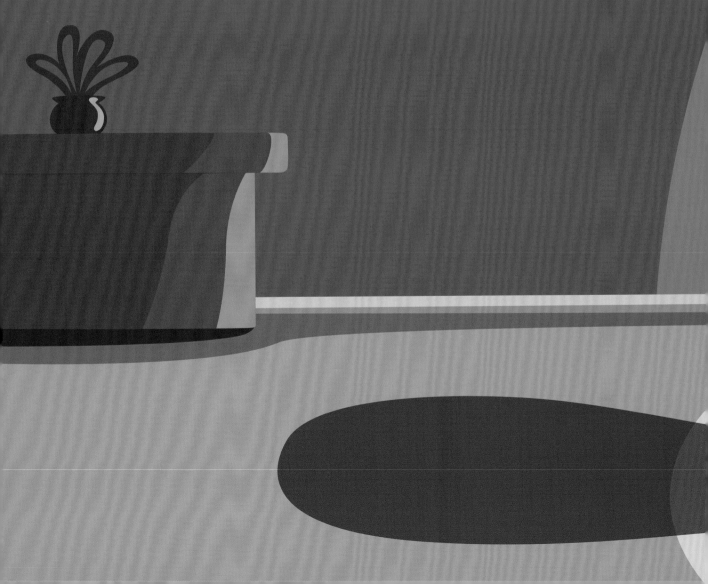

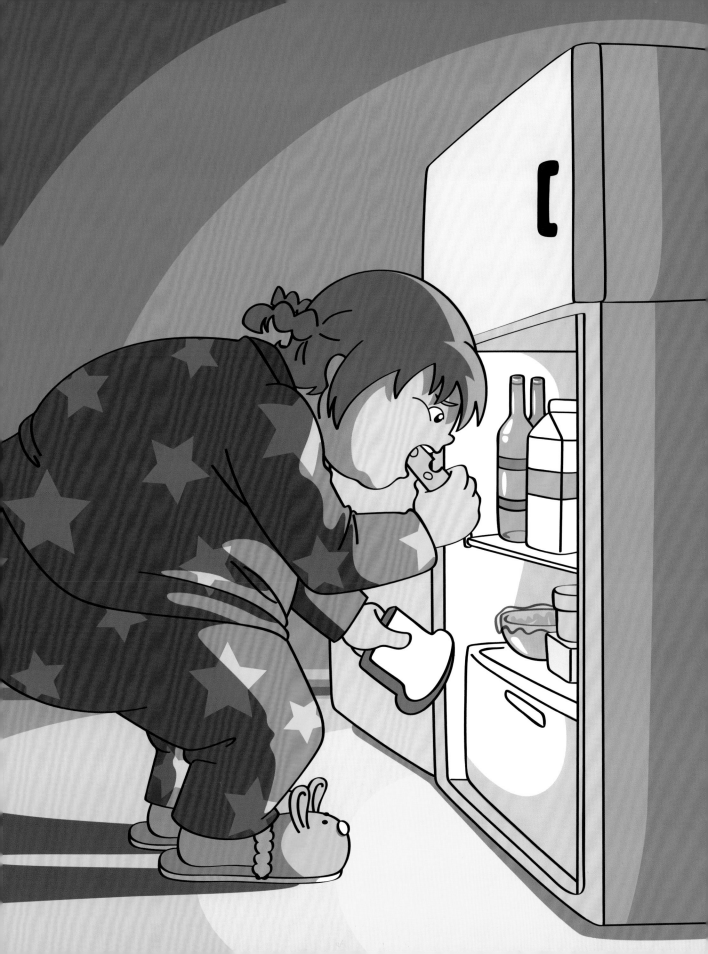

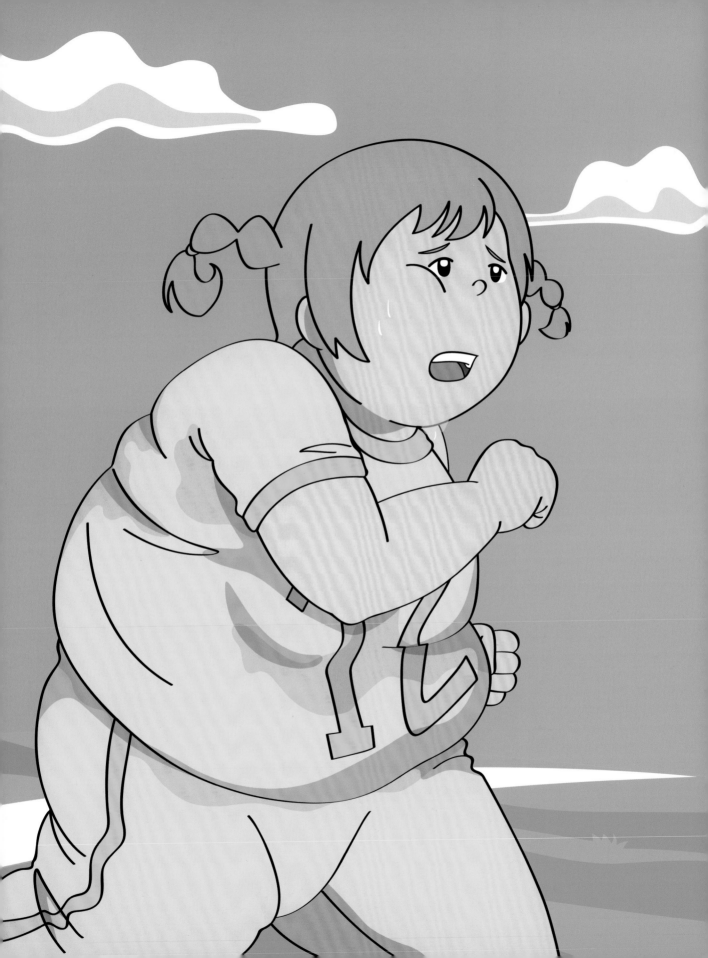

A few weeks later, Maggie was asked to play in a practice
soccer game.
She said yes, although she was terrified of embarrassing herself
and being ashamed.

Maggie couldn't run very fast, but wow, could she kick
that soccer ball.
When she tried running fast she would frequently trip and fall.

Maggie was often out of breath and found it difficult to breathe.
She was also having so much fun she didn't want to leave.

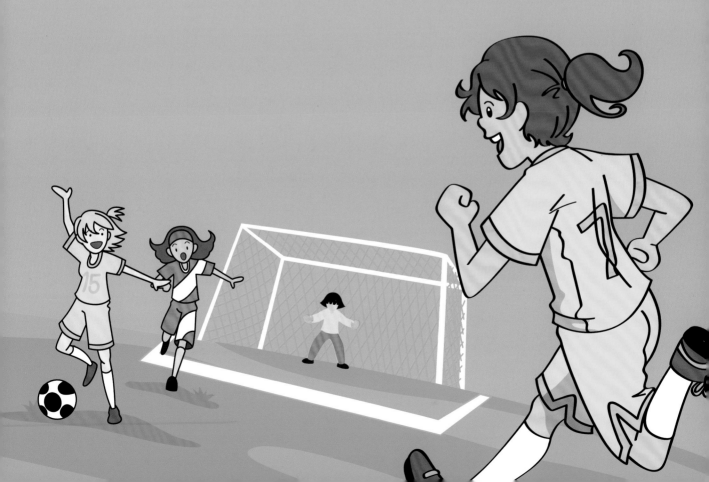

Maggie was frequently teased and made of fun at school.
She was often called fatty and other names that were cruel.

Most of the time Maggie did not wish to respond or counter attack.
Sometimes as much as she tried, she just couldn't hold back.

She told the bullies to stop picking on her, that if she told on them,
it wouldn't be worth the trouble they'd get themselves into.

She said, "Is your life so boring that you have nothing better to do.
How would you like it if someone constantly picked on you?"

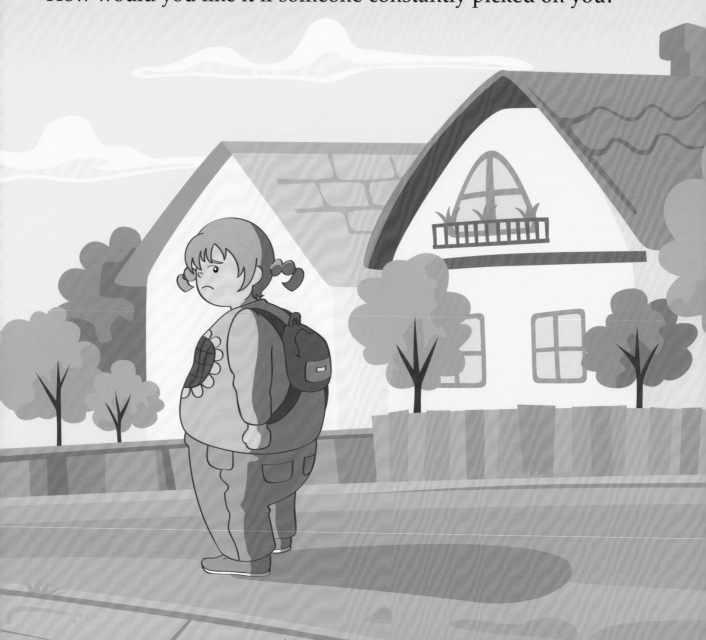

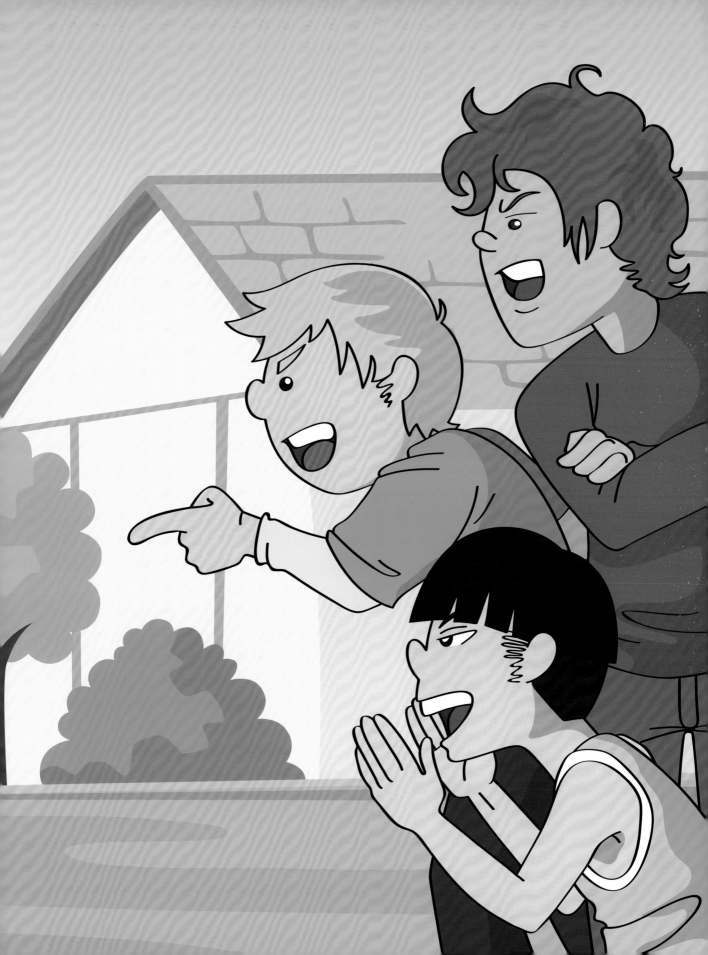

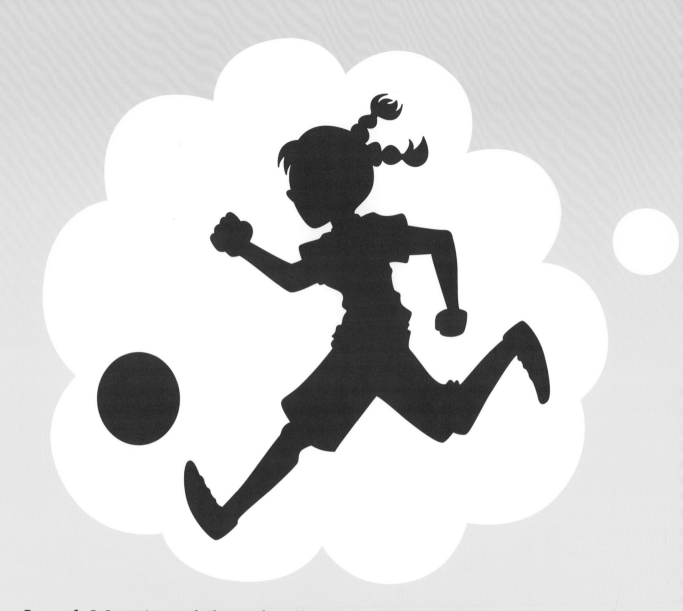

It took Maggie awhile to finally make up her mind.
Maggie really wanted to reduce her stomach and her large behind.

Maggie's parents were happy to support her and Maggie knew
it was not too late.
She also knew she would look better, feel better, and run faster,
if she lost weight.

When was this new way of eating supposed to begin?
"Tomorrow morning," said Maggie, displaying a great big grin.

How long do you think it would take Maggie to become healthier
and trim?

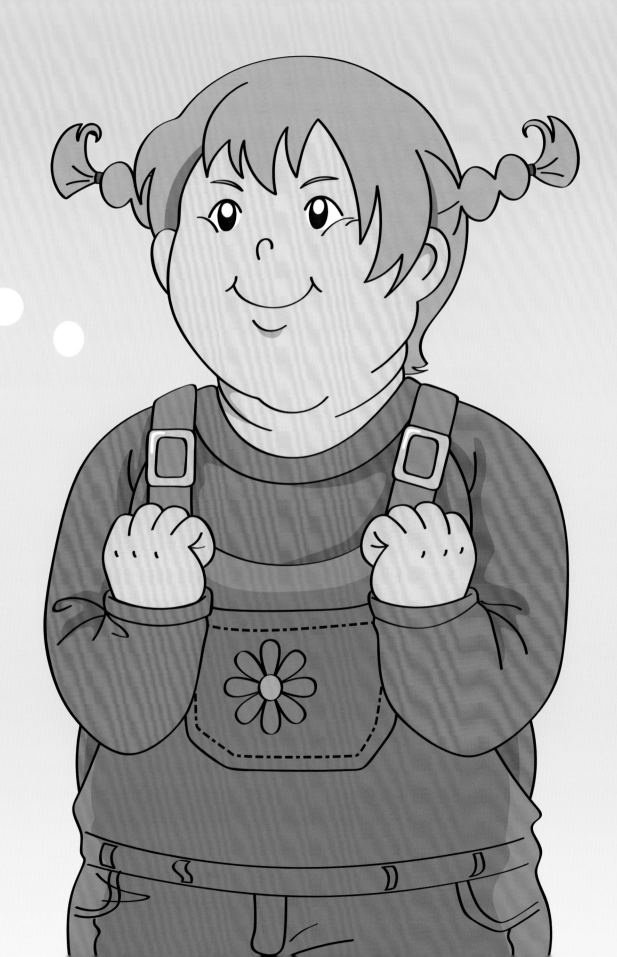

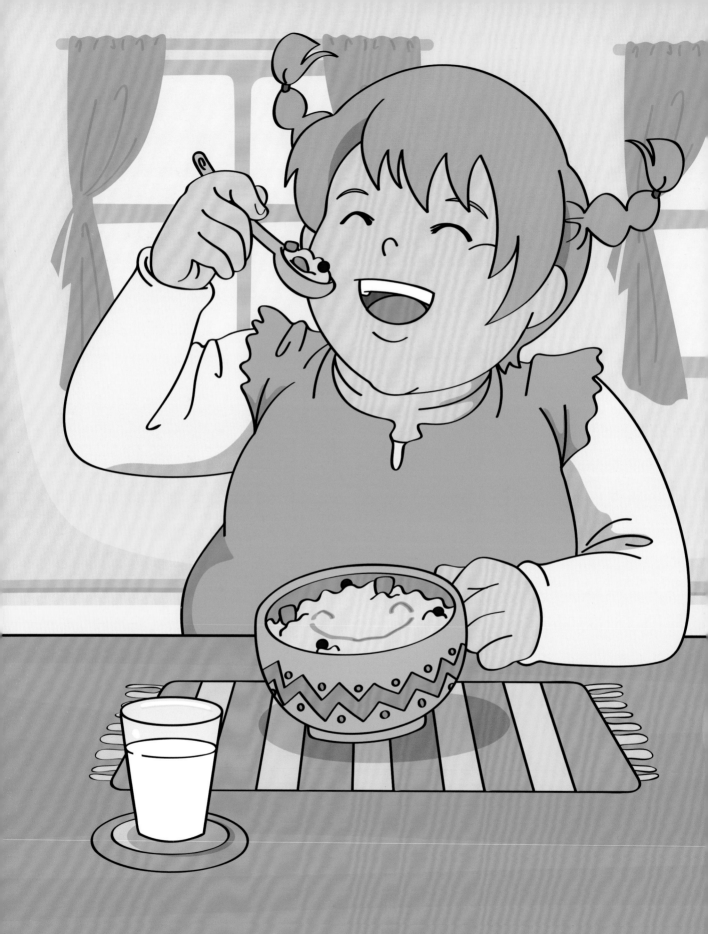

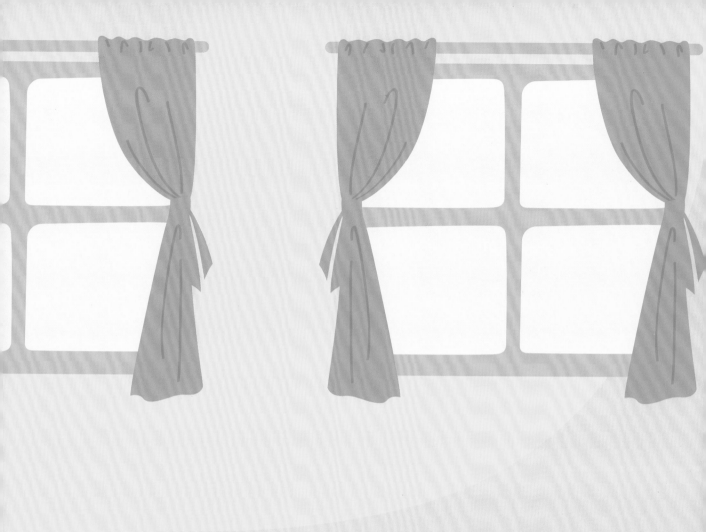

The very next morning Maggie's new lifestyle had begun.
Maggie's plan was to get unhooked from eating unhealthy
foods that she was addicted to, one by one.

Most days' breakfast consisted of oatmeal with yogurt and fruit.
Sometimes Maggie made a smiley face in the bowl which her mom
thought was quite cute.

For lunch Maggie frequently had a turkey sandwich with mustard
and lettuce greens.
For dinner, there were always plenty of vegetables
with various proteins.

Most importantly, Maggie cut out the addictive yummy
tasting in-betweens.

The thought of cutting out junk foods occasionally made Maggie sad.
She was pleasantly surprised that so many healthy foods were quite tasty and for that she was glad.

After the first week, Maggie had lost a small amount of weight.
Bending down and getting up was a little easier which was great.

Maggie still ate plenty of food, but was slowly cutting down on sweets.
She had more energy and was also becoming a better athlete.

Twice a week Maggie allowed herself to have a treat.

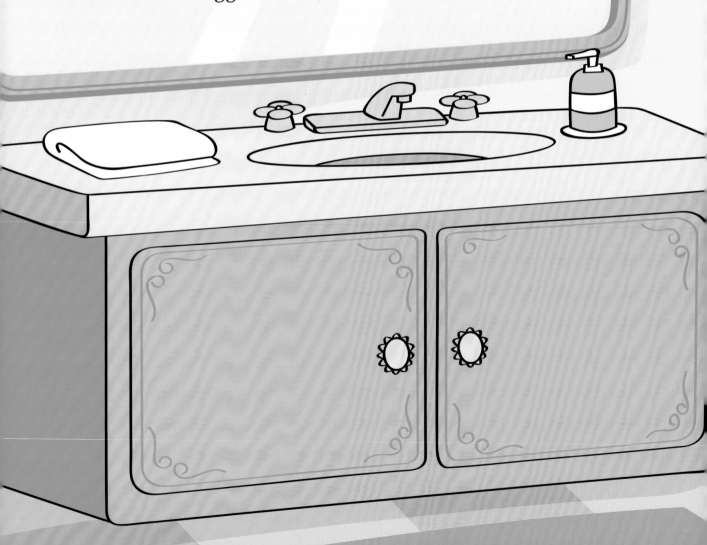

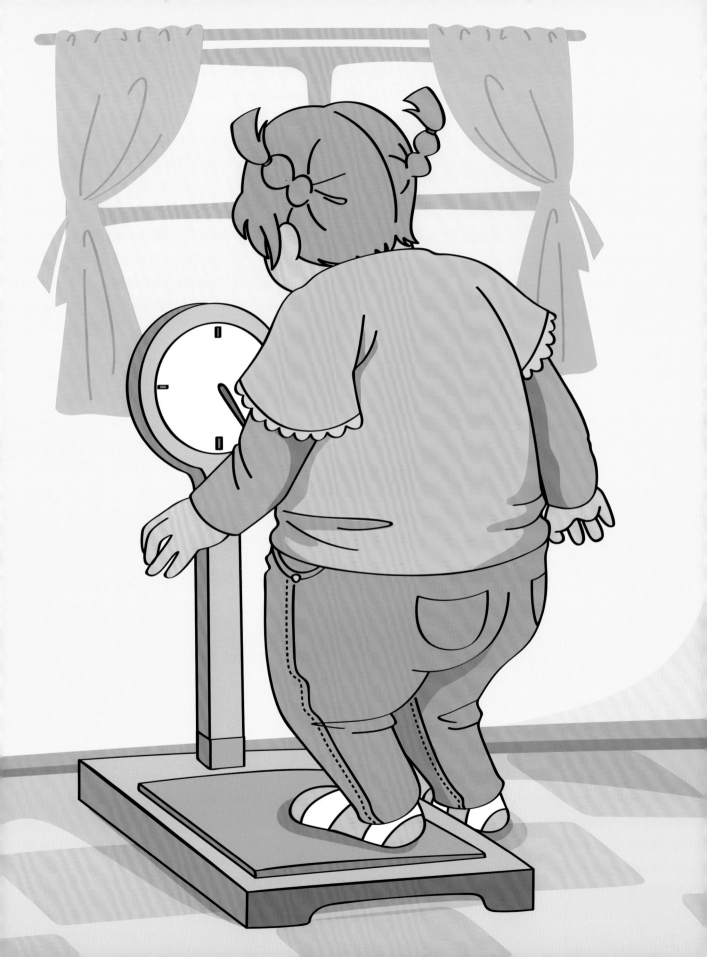

Maggie's baseball team was playing their last game of the year. This time instead of being laughed at, Maggie would soon receive lots of cheer.

Everyone was worried that Maggie would strike out as she did so many times before. No one knew what a special moment Maggie had in store.

There were two outs in the last inning with the game tied one to one. To everyone's surprise and amazement, Maggie hit a home run.

The crowd jumped up and down and roared because their team had finally won.

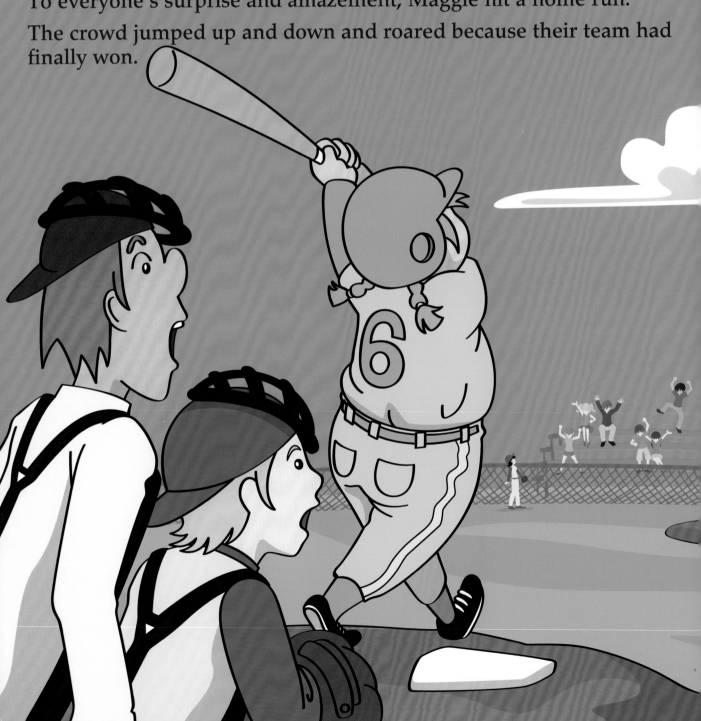

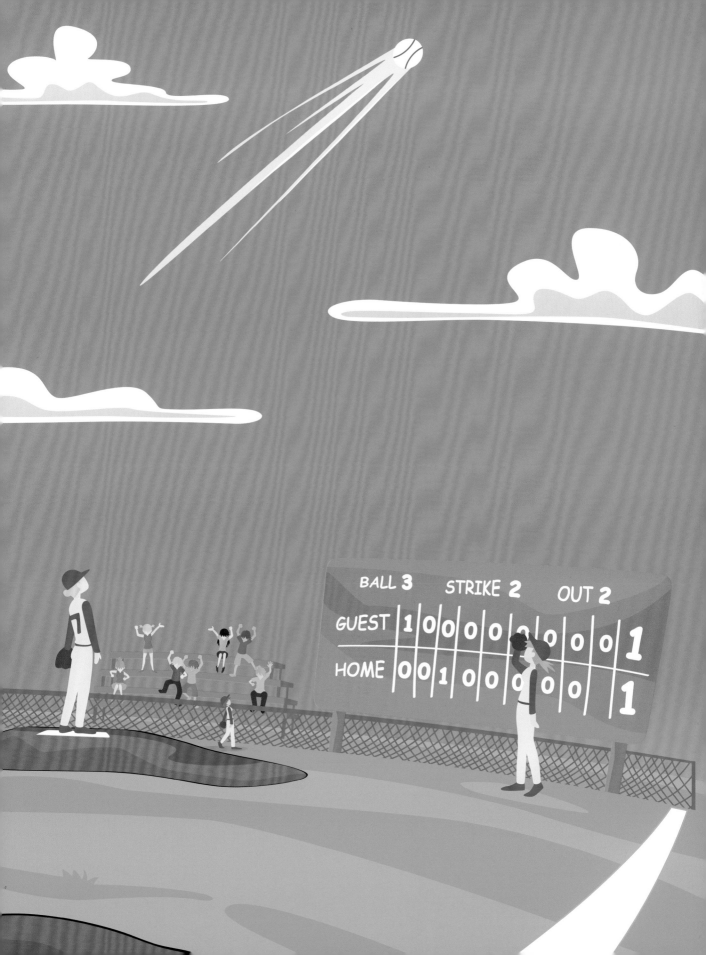

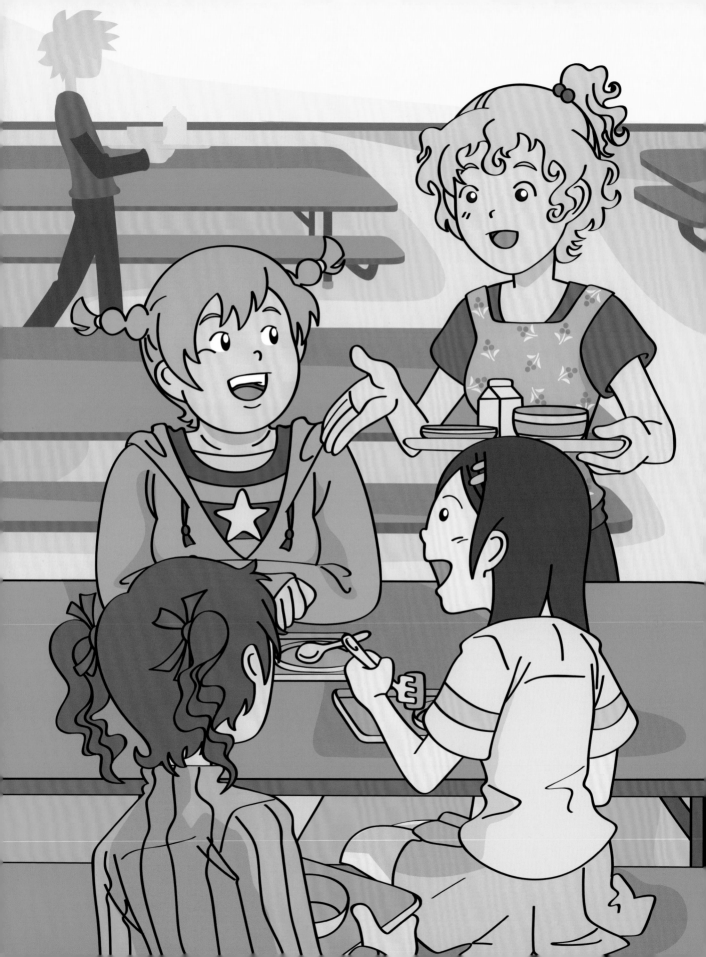

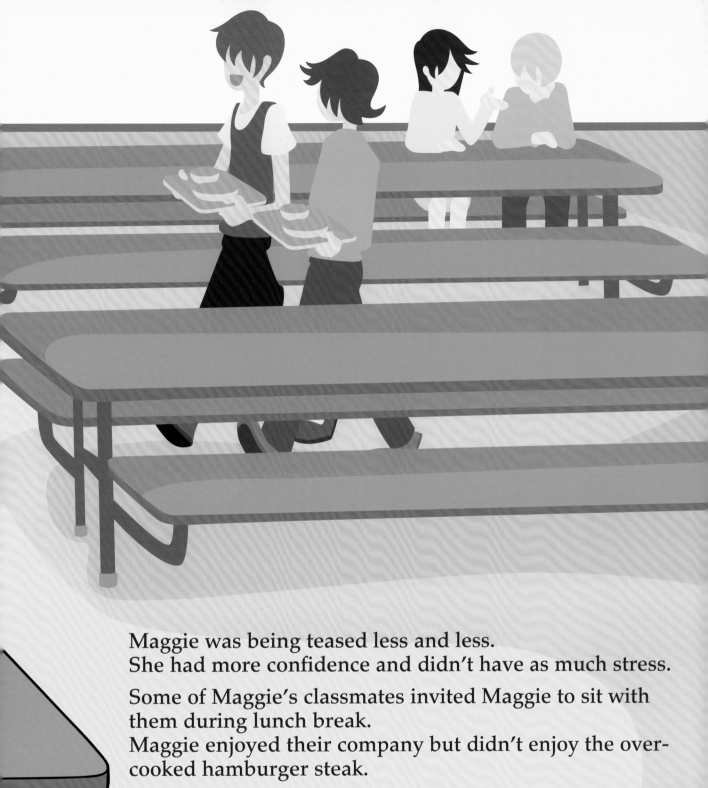

Maggie was being teased less and less.
She had more confidence and didn't have as much stress.

Some of Maggie's classmates invited Maggie to sit with them during lunch break.
Maggie enjoyed their company but didn't enjoy the over-cooked hamburger steak.

They asked Maggie if she wanted to hang out one day.
Maggie said, "Great, sure, I'd love to, okay."

Maggie immediately thought of a great game they all could play.

The following week Maggie was invited to an overnight get together. She was going to Tina's house with Mary, Susan, and Heather.

Maggie couldn't make up her mind on exactly what to pack. Maggie knew she was bringing cut up celery and carrot sticks for snacks.

The girls wanted to know from each other who do you like and who likes you.

Susan and Tina began tickling Maggie saying, "Tell us who, tell us who?"

Maggie giggled and said, "Alright I'll tell you, I like Peter, Robert and Drew."

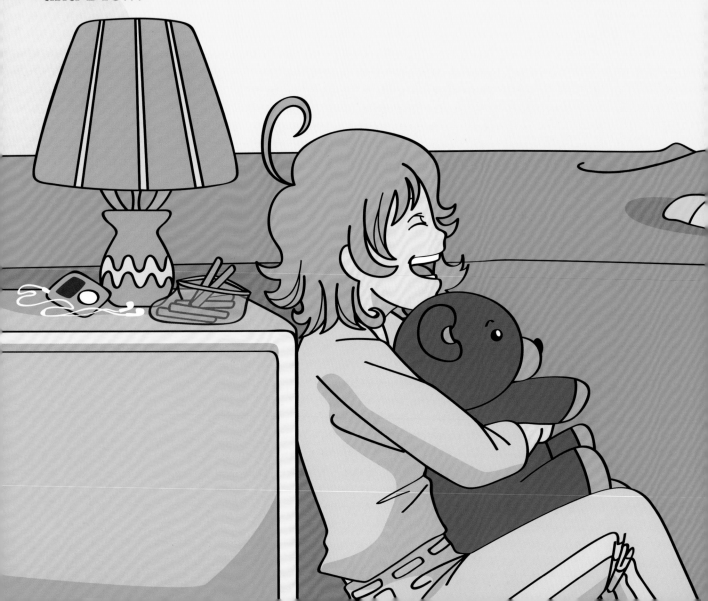

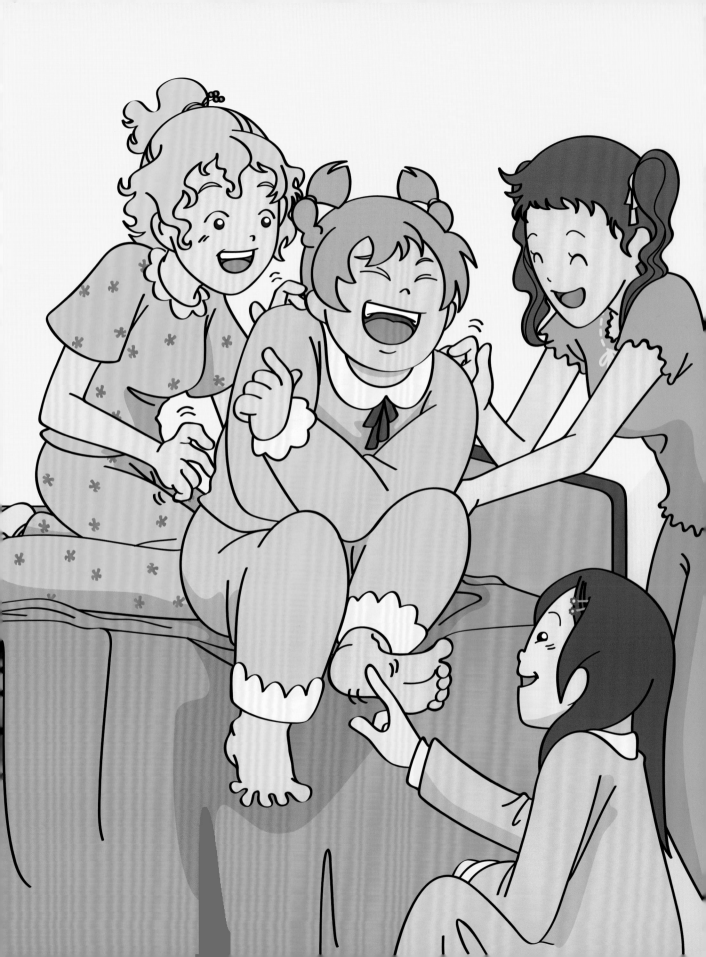

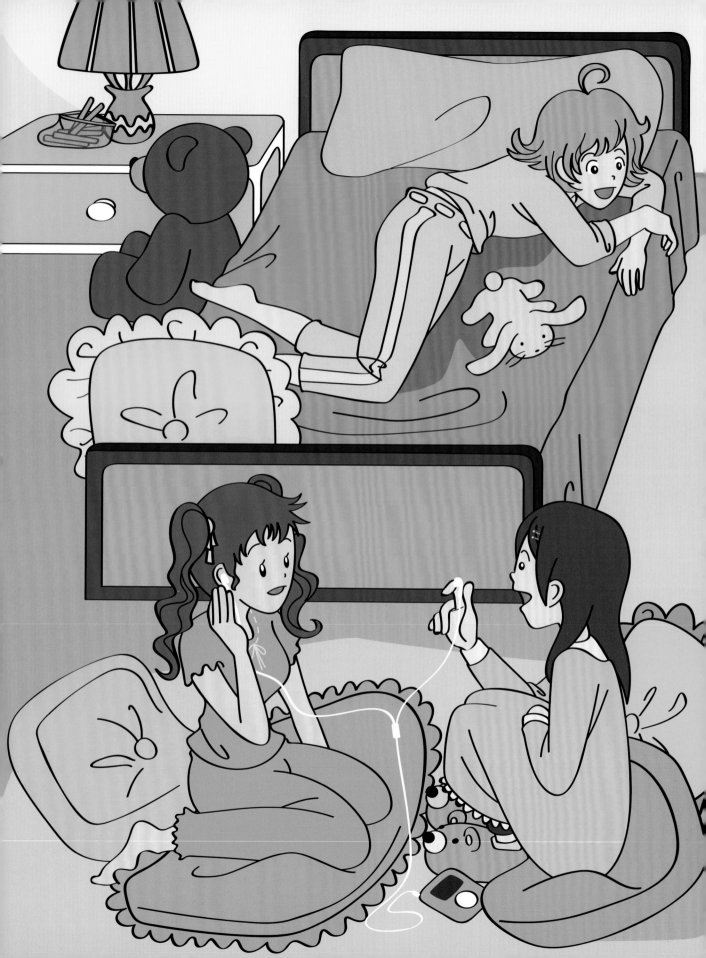

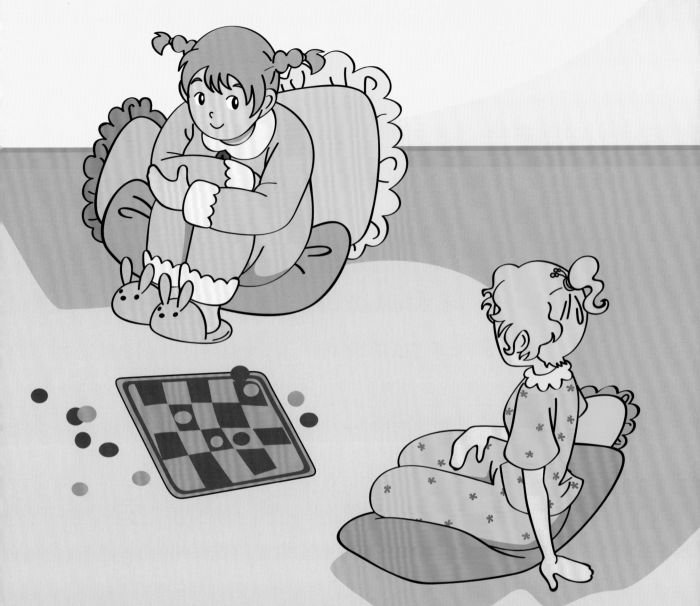

The girls listened to music and also played truth or dare.
Maggie was asked if she believed that being overweight was unfair.

Maggie said, "I realized that I shouldn't eat just because I'm stressed and bored or have nothing better to do."
She also said, "Eating too much junk food is a bad habit that I had gotten myself into."

She told the girls that her doctor suggested that she make better choices in selecting what she eats.
Maggie wanted to play soccer better and was willing to try different vegetables, whole grains and lean meats.

Maggie's mother agreed to cut down on buying addictive treats.

Four months had passed and Maggie was no longer addicted
to junk food and was considerately lighter.
Maggie was healthier and her future looked brighter.

Losing the weight was good for Maggie's health.
She was happier and also proud of herself.

Maggie tried to exercise just about every day.
She was confident that her excess weight was gone to stay.

Maggie's stomach was definitely shrinking and fading away.

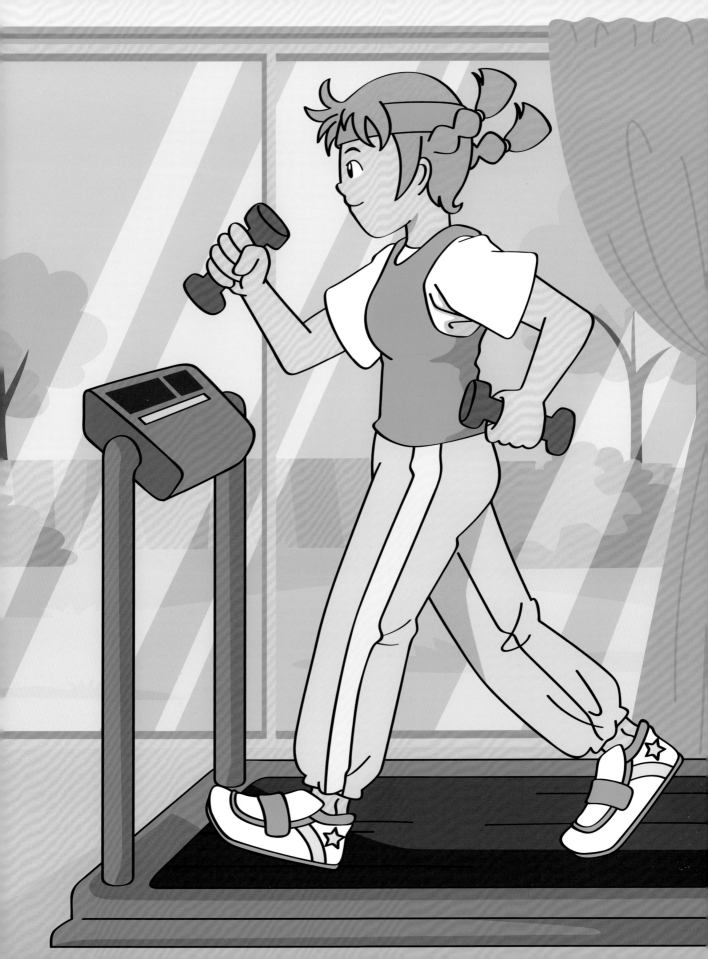

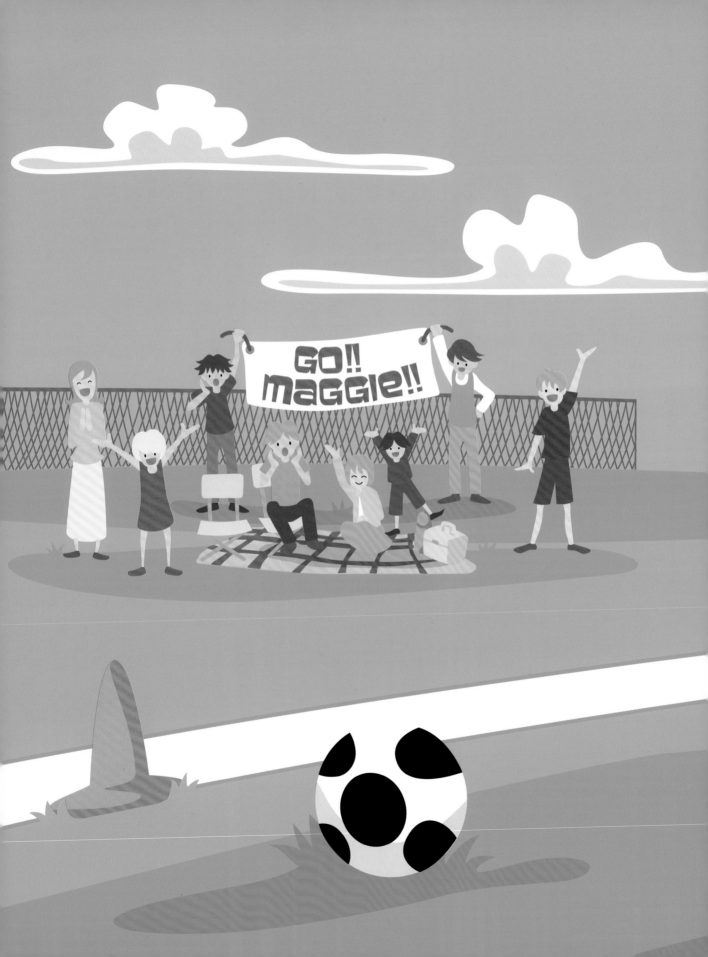

Maggie was now going to soccer practice three to four times a week.
Her team had won their last five games and was on a winning streak.

Maggie was rapidly becoming one of the best players on her team.
Every time Maggie scored a goal, her cheering section would scream.

Maggie looked forward to her Saturday morning game.
More and more people were beginning to know Maggie by name.

Life for Maggie was no longer the same.

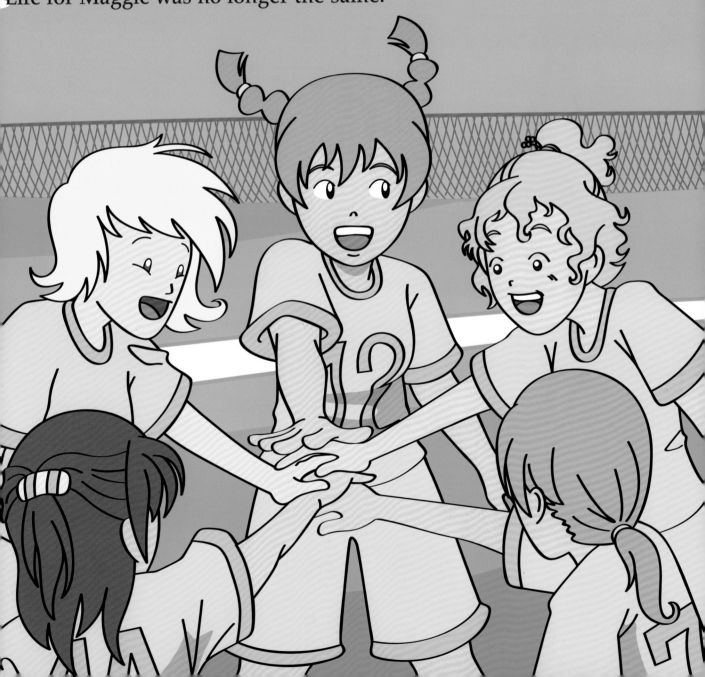

Maggie was starting to get noticed and talked about by some of the gu
Maggie's reputation was slowly increasing and on the rise.

Maggie enjoyed school more and improved on her grades.
With Maggie's added self confidence she was less and less afraid.

Maggie was hoping that her new good fortune was going to last.
She didn't want to return to her less exciting and unhealthier past.

She was so much happier than she used to be and was having a blast.

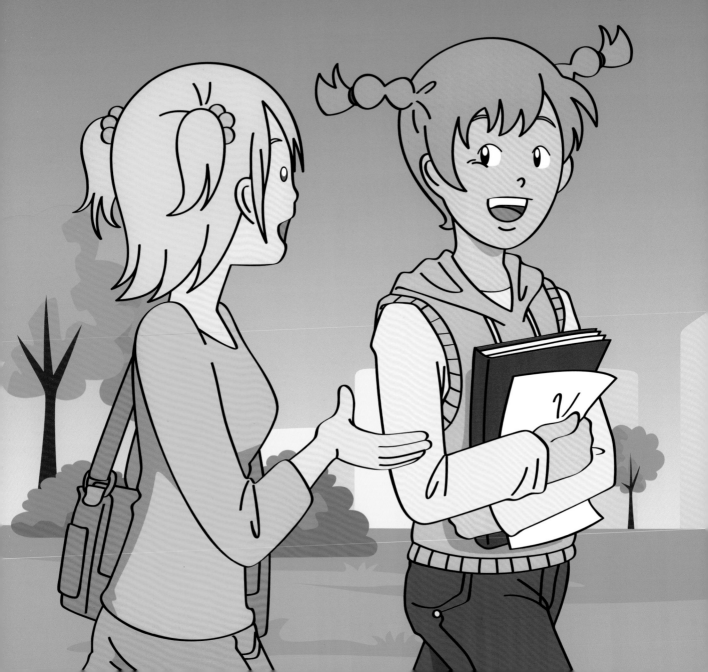

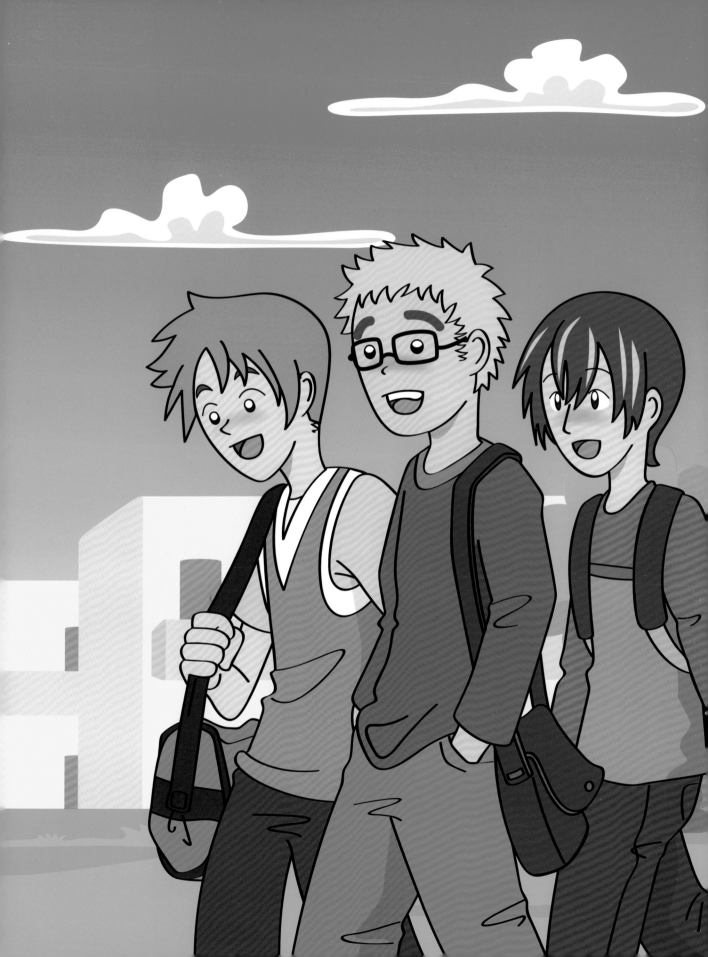

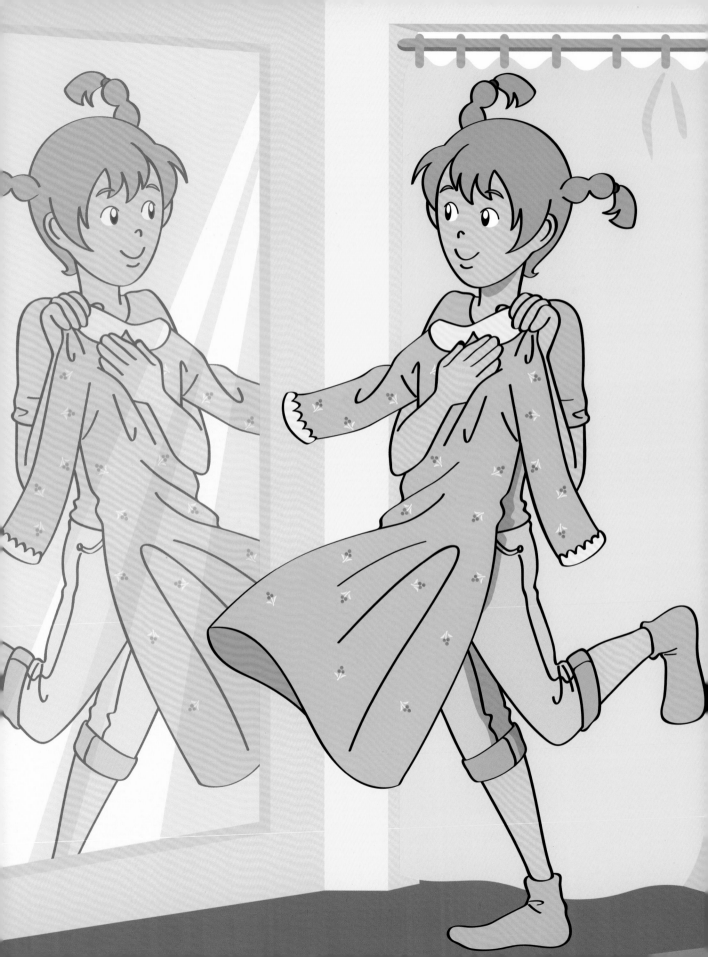

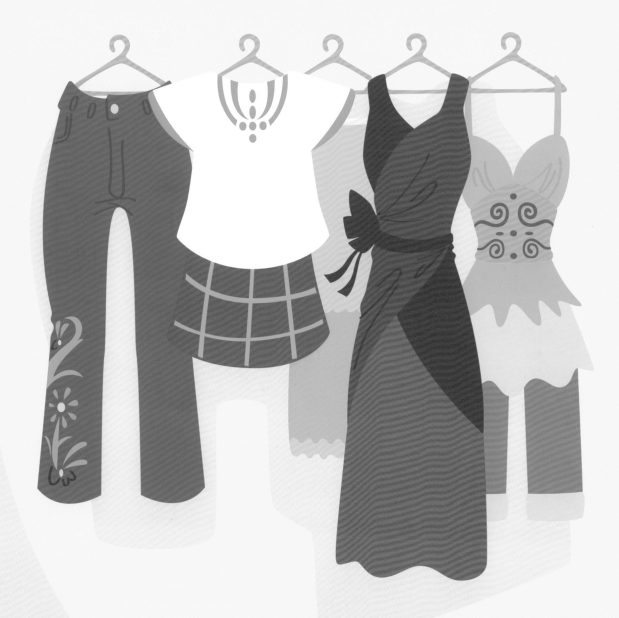

Maggie looked like a different person in her brand new dress.
In a little over ten months Maggie weighed so much less.

All of Maggie's clothes were falling to the floor.
They were so big on her that she couldn't wear them anymore.

Maggie's parents had no choice but to replace all her old clothes.
They had to buy her everything new from her head to her toes.

Maggie was so excited, she felt like she was the star of her own
fashion show.

It was Maggie's last scheduled soccer game of the season.
Maggie's team was in first place and with very good reason.

This game was going to be a good one and any team could win.
Maggie had warmed up for an hour before and was ready to begin.

Maggie's team mate Kyra just missed with a kick that bounced off the upright pole.
Fortunately Maggie was nearby and kicked the ball into the goal.

Maggie and all of her teammates played with their heart and soul.

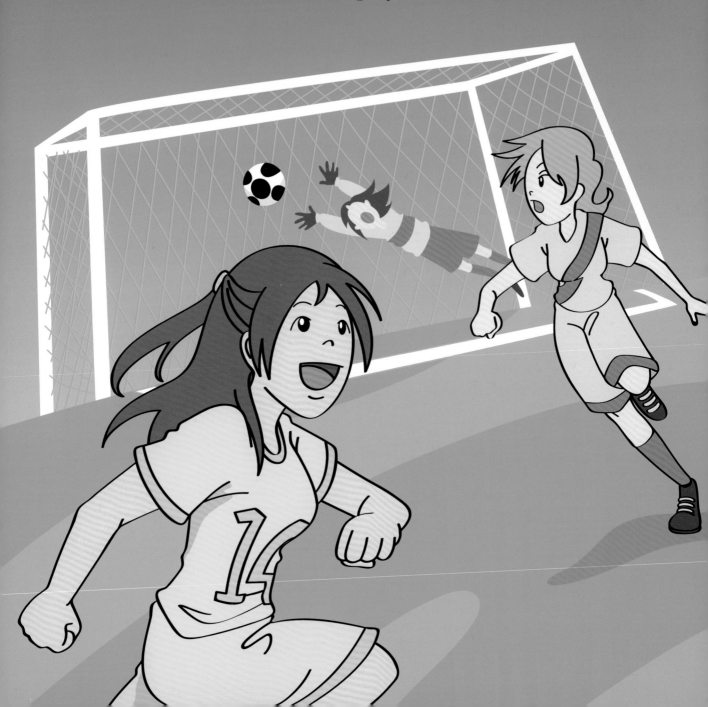

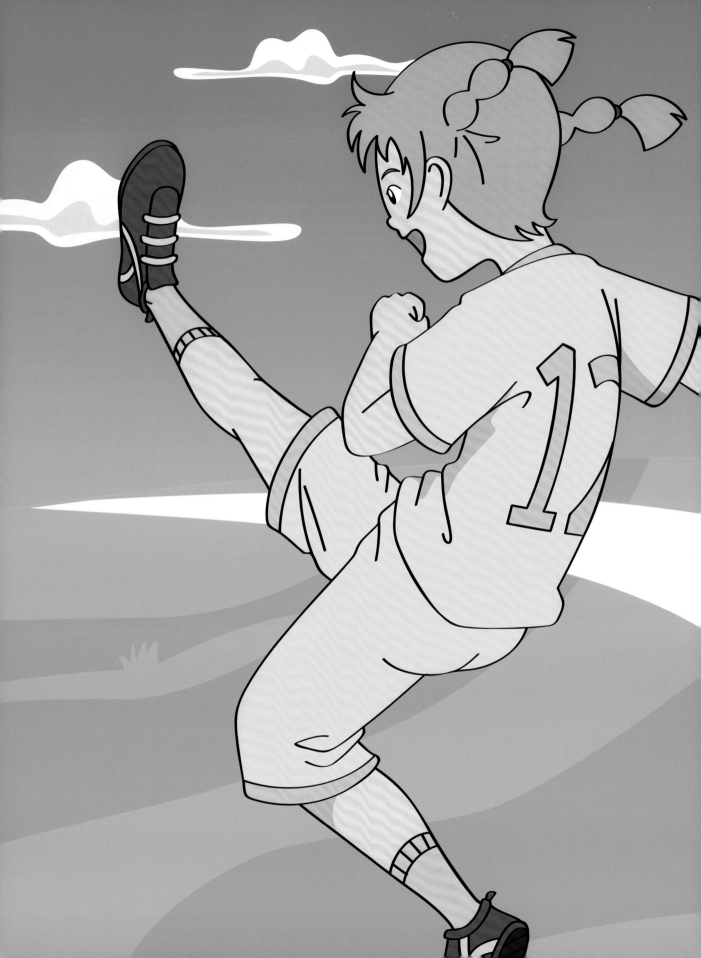

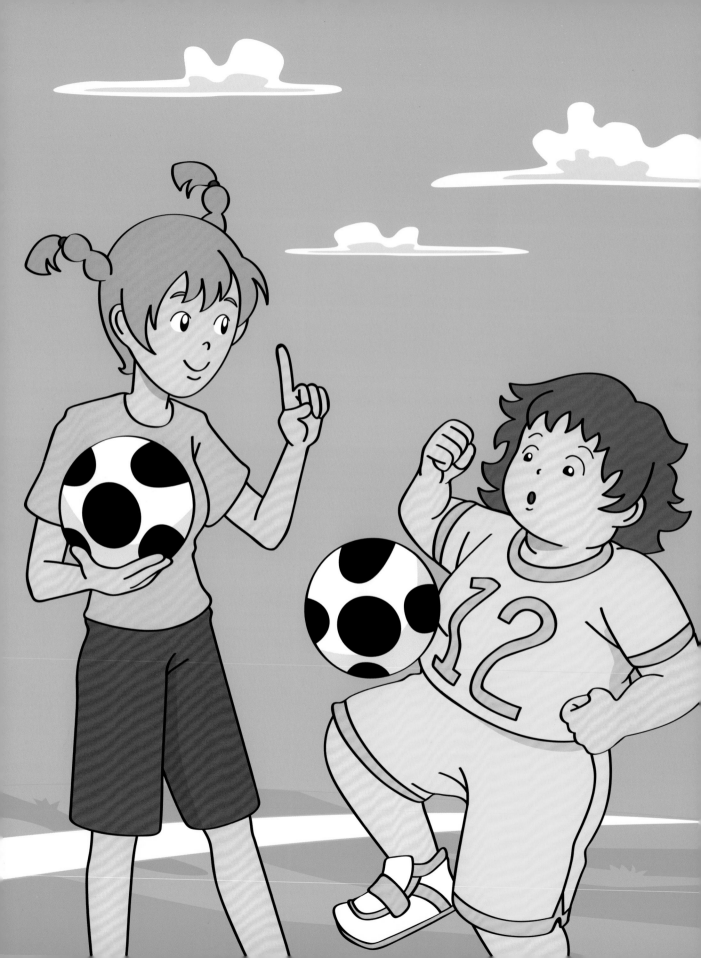

Weeks later Maggie went to the field to practice kicking
her soccer ball.
Maggie was the type that whatever she did she gave it her all.

Practicing in another part of the field was a girl that reminded
Maggie of how she looked a few years ago.
Maggie walked towards that girl and cheerfully said. "Hello."

Maggie introduced herself and the younger girl replied,
"Hi, I'm Kate."
Do you think meeting Kate that day was an act of fate?

Maggie thought that giving Kate a few helpful tips would really
be great.

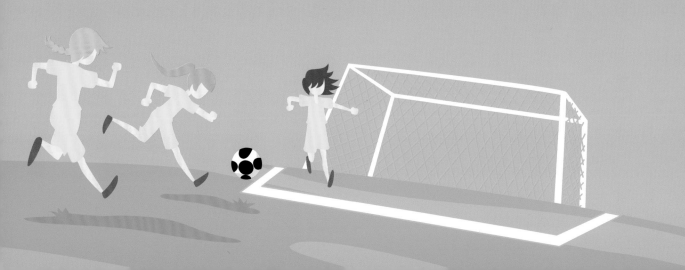

It is sad that people are sometimes judged by how they look.
People shouldn't assume that a pretty cover guarantees a good book.

You should always give people a chance and not judge them until you
see what's in their heart.
It is only then that you will be able to determine what sets them apart.

Now that you're at the end of this book, have you decided what you
are going to do?
Regardless of your current size, eating properly and exercising
regularly will help you become a healthier you.

Helpful hints about what's in the food you eat and how to read
nutrition labels is available at www.nutritiondetectives.com.

Hopefully not the End but a New Beginning!

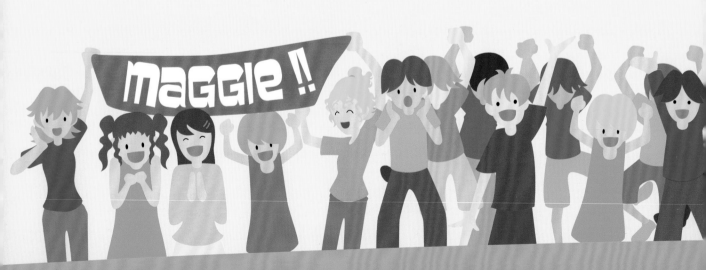

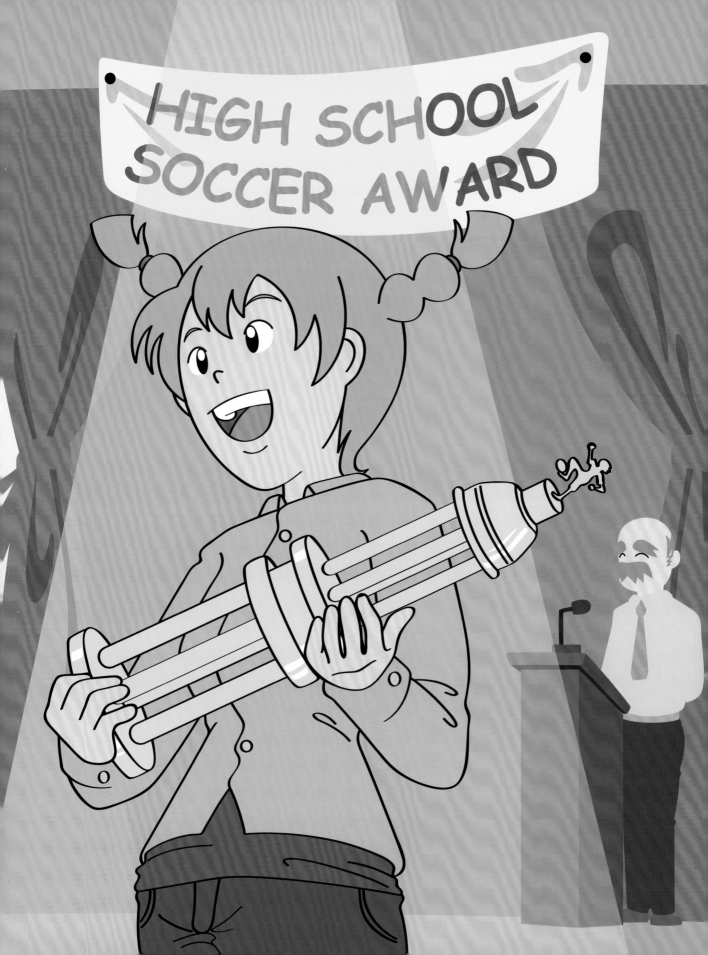

DO IT FOR YOURSELF

Eat only when you're hungry.
Try not to eat late at night.
You are the one you hurt.
Do not eat out of spite.

Do not compete for food,
for to win is to loose.
Do not put your health at risk,
it's up to you to choose.

Do not substitute food for love,
it will only temporarily satisfy you.
You may not understand this compulsive need.
It's destructive and something you should not do.

You deserve to be healthy.
You should try to make the right choice.
By taking more pride in yourself.
Your mind and your body will rejoice.

Paul M Kramer

Other Books Available by Paul M. Kramer

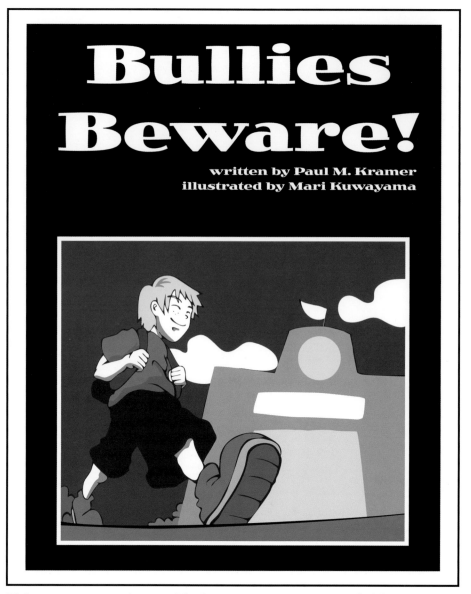

This story was written with the intent to motivate children to seek help when being bullied. Bullying is a very serious problem that has reached unacceptable and uncontrollable levels in recent years and must be dealt with.

Mikey was unwilling to be bullied any longer. Although Mikey was taking karate lessons to learn self-defense, he realized that fighting the bullies was not the best way to solve his problem. Instead, he found the courage to tell his teacher, which turned out to be the right thing to do and as a result the bullies were held accountable for their actions.

This is a must read for children and for the parents of young children who are having problems with bullies and bullying.

ISBN: 978-1-941095-14-0, retail price: $15.95, size: 8" x 10"

Other Books Available by Paul M. Kramer

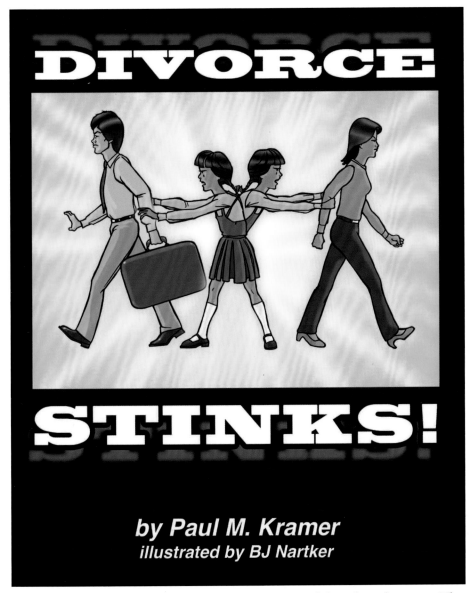

Divorce does stink and changes the lives of families forever. The message for the reader is to realize that the mother and the father are divorcing each other, not their children. They still love their children and it is not the child's fault if their parents get divorced.

ISBN: 0-9819745-4-6, retail price: $15.95, size: 8" x 10"

About the Author

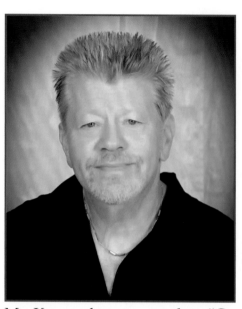

Paul M. Kramer lives in Hawaii on the beautiful island of Maui with his wife Cindy and their son Lukas. Paul was born and raised in New York City.

Mr. Kramer's books attempt to reduce stress and anxiety and resolve important issues children face in their everyday lives. His books are often written in rhyme. They are entertaining, inspirational, educational and easy to read. One of his goals is to increase the child's sense of self worth.

He has written books on various subjects such as bullying, divorce, sleep deprivation, worrying, shyness, and weight issues.

Mr. Kramer has appeared on "Good Morning America," "The Doctors," "CNN Live" as well as several other Television Shows in the United States and Canada. He's been interviewed and aired on many radio programs including the British Broadcasting System and has had countless articles written about his work in major newspapers and magazines throughout the world.

More information about this book and Paul M. Kramer's other books are available on his website at www.alohapublishers.com.